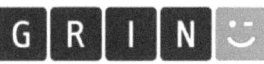

Bibliographic information published by the German National Library:

The German National Library lists this publication in the National Bibliography; detailed bibliographic data are available on the Internet at http://dnb.dnb.de .

Imprint:

Copyright © 2013 GRIN Verlag
Print and binding: Books on Demand GmbH, Norderstedt Germany
ISBN: 9783668670976

This book at GRIN:

https://www.grin.com/document/212604

Cosmas Alfred Butele

A Survey of the Species Composition, Distribution and Relative Abundance of Tsetseflies (Diptera: Glossinidae) of Adjumani District, North Western Uganda

GRIN Verlag

GRIN - Your knowledge has value

Since its foundation in 1998, GRIN has specialized in publishing academic texts by students, college teachers and other academics as e-book and printed book. The website www.grin.com is an ideal platform for presenting term papers, final papers, scientific essays, dissertations and specialist books.

Visit us on the internet:

http://www.grin.com/

http://www.facebook.com/grincom

http://www.twitter.com/grin_com

BUTELE COSMAS ALFRED

BASIC TSETSE FLY SPECIES IDENTIFICATION AND DISTRIBUTION
ANALYSIS TECHNIQUES

*A Survey of the Species Composition, Distribution and Relative
Abundance of Tsetseflies (Diptera: Glossinidae) of Adjumani District,
North Western Uganda.*

ATLANTIC INTERNATIONAL UNIVERSITY
HONOLULU, HAWAII

© 02/04/2013.

ABSTRACT

Adjumani District, located in the northwestern part of Uganda, has had a long history of tsetse and trypanosomiasis. However, tsetse control methods and operations in the district were being guided by mere number and location of sleeping sickness cases treated in Adjumani Hospital and complaints of tsetse infestation received from the villages, without reference to precise knowledge of the particular tsetse species present, their distribution and relative abundance. It was thought that only one riverine tsetse fly species existed in the district. Accordingly only one tsetse control method of tsetse trapping using insecticide treated pyramidal traps meant for riverine tsetse was being promoted in the district. A systematic tsetse survey was therefore planned to establish the particular tsetse species present in the district. 7 locations (parishes) were first selected for a preliminary area-wide tsetse survey, basing on number and location of sleeping sickness cases treated in Adjumani Hospital. The preliminary survey was then carried out in the 7 selected locations (parishes) to determine trapping sites. 10 pyramidal traps were deployed at a distance of 250m apart along river banks in each village in the location, and checked (milked) after 72 hours (3 days). A total of 220 pyramidal traps were used. Six locations found to have tsetse flies were considered as study locations. Two villages were selected as trapping sites in each of the 6 study locations on the basis of high baseline fly trapping density (FTD) or species complexity, giving a total of 12 trapping sites. FTD was calculated as the number of flies caught per trap per day. Routine trapping in the trapping sites took 6 months from April to September 2002. Three pyramidal traps and 3 biconical traps were deployed, spaced 50m apart in each trapping site to catch adult tsetse flies, and checked after every 24 hours (1 day), once a week, giving a total of 24 samples for each trapping site. Tsetse fly species caught were identified using external morphological features. The survey revealed that at least 3 different species of tsetse flies exist in the district: *Glossina fuscipes fuscipes*, *G. morsitans*, and *G. pallidipes*. *G. f. fuscipes* was the most abundant species distributed in all the 6 parishes and 12 trapping sites with an average fly trapping density (FTD) of 1.765, followed by *G. m. submorsitans* found in Maaji-Sinyanya-Ofu Village in Ukusijoni Parish, Okawa Village in Palaro Parish and Pakwinya Village in Odu Parish with an average FTD of 0.174 and the least abundant species being *G. Pallidipes* confined to Maaji-Sinyanya-Ofu Village in Ukusijoni Parish, with an average FTD of 0.0308. In total 1,570 tsetse flies were caught during the survey period which disaggregated into 635 males (40%), 935 females (60%). There were 416 non-teneral male tsetse flies (26%) and 219 teneral male tsetse flies (14%), 637 non-teneral female tsetse flies (41%) and 298 teneral female tsetse flies (19%). During the survey period, a total of 41 Sleeping Sickness cases from the 6 study locations (parishes) was being treated in Adjumani Hospital, which disaggregated into 6 Sleeping Sickness stage I cases (1 male national 2.4%, 2 female nationals 4.8%, 3 male refugees and other people from Southern Sudan 7.3%, 0 female refugees and other people from Southern Sudan 00%), and 35 Sleeping Sickness stage II cases (6 male nationals 14.6%, 2 female nationals 4.8 %, 8 male refugees and other people from Southern Sudan 19.5%, 19 female refugees and other people from Southern Sudan 46.3%). This information on the three different tsetse species present and their distribution pattern in the district should now be used to guide choice of species specific tsetse control methods in future.

2

TABLE OF CONTENTS

LIST OF FIGURES

LIST OF ACRONYMS

COCTU   Coordinating Office for Control of Trypanosomiasis in Uganda

FAO   Food and Agriculture Organization of the United Nations

FTD   Fly Trapping Density

Km^2 Kilometres squared

m   metres

MAAIF   Ministry of Agriculture, Animal Industry and Fisheries (of Uganda)

MOH   Ministry of Health

MSF   Medicine Sans Frontiers

pers.comm.   personal communication

PhD   Doctor of Philosophy

INTRODUCTION

Adjumani District, formerly called East Moyo County of the neighbouring Moyo District, is located in north western Uganda, $2^0 53$"N to $3^0 37$"N and $31^0 24$"E to $32^0 4$"E in the west Nile Region, lying on the low plateau at an altitude of 9000-1500m above sea level (Rwabwoogo, 1998). It is bordered on the north and west by Moyo District, in the northeast by the Southern Sudan and on east and South by Gulu District and on the Southwest by Arua and Yumbe districts. The district has an area of 3,128 Km^2 (Anonymous, 2002a-unpublished). Dratele (1999) suggested the established climate of the area comprising of two seasons –one rainy season (March –October) and dry season (November-March), although recently the rainfall pattern has become unreliable. There is also a short dry spell in the area in the month of June. The rainfall in the area would normally range from 750 to 1250mm per annum (Rwabwoogo, 1998). The district is general flat and hot especially during dry season (Anonymous, 2000a). It is blessed with a number of water bodies, namely rivers Itirikwa, Esia, Adidi, Tete, Surumu, Odraji and many other seasonal streams, and one forest reserve-Zoka forest (Dratele, 1999). The district is extensive savanna grassland with scattered woodlands and thickets (Rwabwoogo, 1998). The vegetation may be classed into woodlands, moist *Combretum* savanna and a mosaic of *Butyrospemum* savanna and dry *Combretum* savannas (Langdale-Brown, *et al.*, 1964). It has a variety of wild animals such as buffaloes, antelopes, hippopotami, dikes, warthogs, baboons, monkeys, and crocodiles. The human population of Adjumani District by 2002 comprised Southern Sudan refugees and Ugandan nationals. The lot of refugees stood at 70,000 people compared to that of nationals, 130,000, totaling to 200,000 (Anonymous, 2002a-unpublished). Agricultural economic activities carried out in the district include fish farming, cultivation of crops such as simsim, maize, millet, soybeans, etc.; planting of trees such as neem and teak (Rwabwoogo, 1998; and Egadu, 2000-unpublished), rearing of livestock such as cattle, goats, sheep, poultry (Anonymous, 2002b-unpublished). By 2002, the district had 12 sub counties, 34 parishes, and 134 villages. Adjumani District is part of a bigger tsetse and trypanosomiasis bane, in Uganda and Africa in general. Sleeping sickness has been reported in 37 sub-Saharan African countries (Biryomumaisho, 2007; and Science Daily, 2012), including Uganda. According to MAAIF (2012), about 70% of Uganda is tsetse infested ($140,000km^2$), including Adjumani District. The problem of tsetse and trypanosomiasis Adjumani District could have started time immemorial, but the first known recorded history dates back to 1912 when the Christian Missionaries first came to the area (Dratele, 1999). Tsetse and Sleeping Sickness broke-out originating from Boroli Village in Palaro Parish, Pakelle Sub County. The settlers there were forced to leave the place. The missionaries who settled in the neighboring Indriani Village were also forced to leave for Pakelle and Moyo and built missions in Pakelle and Moyo respectively, which stand up to today. Before this escape took place, the first priest in the place Reverend Father Molinario died and was buried in Indriani Village where a monument

7

stands in the abundant place up to today (Drasi Saverio, pers.comm. 2002). Under the then British colonial government, an office for tsetse control was established in the area in 1940, headed by a man called Ogayi. The main methods used were bush clearing, live bait technology, and insecticide spraying on tree trunks and branches. A health centre was also set up in the area in 1945 and a medical team was deployed to treat Sleeping Sickness cases. With the tsetse control and medical teams both actively involved, the tsetse and Sleeping Sickness outbreak was brought under control in 1947 (Drasi Saverio, pers.comm. 2002). In 1968, after independence, tsetse control team was redeployed with the bush clearing and spraying sections to expand areas for human settlement and cultivation (Drasi Saverio, pers.comm. 2002). Since then Sleeping Sickness was only heard of but not seen by the young generation in the area until after 1980 (Drici Eusebio, pers.comm. 2002). The insurgency of 1980 forced many residents of the area to take refuge in Southern Sudan and those who never ran to Southern Sudan gathered in trading centers and churches, leaving the village vacant. The area was over grown by bush and encroached again by bush and wild animals. This gave an opportunity for the tsetse vector population to rise and spread to areas previously reclaimed. While in Southern Sudan people were exposed to high Sleeping Sickness infection. In 1986, many people returned from exile infected with trypanosomiasis in their blood and became exposed to the high number of tsetse flies already waiting in their home areas. The high number of tsetse flies helped to fasten the spread of Sleeping Sickness and this resulted into another epidemic in 1991. Medicine Sans Frontiers (MSF) France came in the district to reduce the provenience by mass screening of the community and treating the patients for Sleeping Sickness in September 1991 (MSF France, 1992; and COCTU, 1995). The Department of Entomology which was already operational in the area was also strengthened further to reduce the vector population. It mobilized the local leaders of high-risk areas and provided them with tsetse traps (Dratele, 1999). The situation eventually subsided. In 1996, yet another Sleeping Sickness epidemic was reported in the area (COCTU, 1996) which was later controlled. Between 1999 and 2001, the prevalence of trypanosomiasis in the district was observed to be on the rise again (Dratele, 1999 and MOH, 2001). The prevalence of bovine trypanosomiasis alone in the district stood at 36.4% (Dratele, 1999). From October 1999 to March 2000, a total of 64 Sleeping Sickness patients had been undergoing treatment in Adjumani Hospital, 13 of them (20%) were Southern Sudanese, 16 (25%) Southern Sudanese refugees living in various settlement camps in the district, and 35 (55%) were Ugandans from within Adjumani and Gulu districts (Anonymous, 2000b-unpublished). There was another outbreak of Sleeping Sickness reported in the area in 2001 (Mutumba-Lule, 2001). The situation was complicated by uncontrolled movement of Southern Sudanese refugees from and to the neighboring southern Sudan where trypanosomiasis had reached epidemic proportions (Hursey, 2001). Yet, there was no tsetse and trypanosomiasis control in Southern Sudan owing to the 20-year old civil war there by then. Health officials had warned that if the

8

situation in Northwestern Uganda was not arrested, the disease could spread to other areas (Mutumba-Lule, 2001). It was even more worrying that there were increasing numbers of melarsoprol drug resistance among Sleeping Sickness patients reported in the area in 2001 (Barett, 2001). There was also corresponding increase in the numbers of the vector tsetse flies in the district recorded earlier in 2000 (Anonymous, 2000c-unpublished). Active (outreach) Sleeping Sickness sensitization and screening programmes by MSF (France) ended around the same time. All along it was thought that only one riverine tsetse fly species existed in the district. Accordingly only one tsetse control method of using insecticide treated pyramidal traps designed specifically to trap riverine tsetse was being promoted in the district. This, systematic, tsetse survey establishes the particular tsetse species present and their distribution patterns in the district, to inform the process of tsetse control planning, the choice of control methods to use, and stop wastage of resources.

Table 1: The Tsetse Fly Survey Study Locations (Parishes) and Trapping Sites (Villages) in Adjumani District, April – September 2002

Sub county	Study Location (Parishes)	Trapping Sites (Villages)
1. Adropi	1. Paridi	1. Esia
		2. Moinya
2. Ciforo	2. Ukusijoni	3. Panyewe – Kobo
		4. Maaji – Sinyanya - Ofu
3. Ofua	3. Odu	5. Odu
		6. Pakwinya
4. Pakele	4. Ataboo	7. Paluga
		8. Palanyua
	5. Palaro	9. Okawa
		10.Melijo
5. Dzaipi	6. Arinyapi	11.Madulu/Itoasi
		12.Nzolohwe/Oniazo

MATERIALS AND METHODS

The materials used include pyramidal traps, biconical traps, fly cages, Canada balsam, entomological boxes and pins, compound microscope, microscope slides and cover slips, naphthalene, labels, stationery, camera (Kodak), panga knives, ethyl acetate, and x10 hand lenses. 7 locations (Parishes) were selected for a preliminary area-wide tsetse survey, basing on number and location of Sleeping Sickness cases treated in Adjumani Hospital from October 1999 to march 2000 (Anonymous, 2000b-unpublished). The preliminary survey was carried out from July 2001 to January 2002 in the 7 selected locations (parishes) to determine trapping sites. 10 pyramidal traps were deployed at a distance of 250m apart along riverbanks in each village in the location, and checked (milked) after 72 hours (3 days). A total of 220 pyramidal traps were used. One location (parish) was found not to have tsetse flies and was dropped. The other six locations were found to have tsetse flies and were then considered as study locations. Two villages were

9

selected as trapping sites in each of the 6 study locations on the basis of high baseline fly trapping density (FTD) or species complexity, giving a total of 12 trapping sites (Table 1). FTD is the number of flies caught per trap per day. Routine trapping in the trapping sites took 6 months from April 2002 to September 2002. Three pyramidal traps and 3 biconical traps were deployed, spaced 50 m apart in each trapping site to catch adult tsetse flies, and checked after every 24 hours (1 day), once a week giving a total of 24 samples for each trapping site. The tsetse flies caught were distinguished from other similar biting flies using the method described by FAO (1982a). Tsetse species caught were identified using external morphological features as described by Smart, et al. (1943), Nash (1969), FAO (1982a) and Cook (1996). Each species of tsetse identified were recorded against the trap number and type of vegetation from which it was collected. Vegetation in each trapping site has been described using the dominant woody species, trees and shrubs, following from Langdale-Brown, et al. (1964). Teneral and non-teneral flies were recognized using the method described by FAO (1982b). Tsetse flies caught were also sexed by observing the ventral surface of the genitalia under the microscope, as described by Nash (1969), and FAO (1982b); presence of hypopygium shows that the tsetse fly is male while the absence shows it is female. FTD was calculated for each trapping site, pooled for each study location and the whole district. Any tsetse fly caught, if still alive, was killed by using ethyl acetate, a method described by FAO (1982b). After having been killed with the killing agent, a number of each species identified was pinned using entomological pins as described by Service (1980) and placed in an entomological box for future reference. Important external diagnostic parts of each tsetse species identified were mounted on microscope slides using the method described by FAO (1982b), drawn and documented for training new tsetse control personnel and to help guide tsetse control personnel to easily identify tsetse species encountered in the field. Naphthalene was placed in the entomological box to prevent the specimens from being eaten by cockroaches, ants, mites and other scavengers and from attack by fungi. All specimens whether pinned in entomological box or mounted on microscope slides have been labeled with the data in pencil as described by Service (1980). Records of fly catches were used to assess the spatial distribution and relative abundance by number of tsetse species at each trapping site and location. Fly catch data were analyzed using the computer program of SPSS 10.1 for Windows. Catch data for female and male flies in each trapping site were analyzed separately. Fly catches were also compared between different trapping sites to assess location effects. Chi-square was used to analyze teneral males, non-teneral males, teneral females and non-teneral females. To compare relative abundance and distribution of the different tsetse species between study locations, each set of data from the traps at different trapping sites were pooled and compared between locations. Results in the following section have been presented in form of tables, graphs and charts.

RESULTS AND DISCUSSIONS

In the preliminary survey using pyramidal traps only, two tsetse fly species were identified: *Glossina fuscipes fuscipes* of *Palpalis* group and very few individuals of *Morsitans* species group (Table II). This provided the baseline information for selecting study locations (parishes) and trapping sites (villages).

Table II: Results of Preliminary Tsetse Survey

Location (Parish)	Trapping Site (Village)	Tsetse Flies Caught	Fly Trapping Density (FTD)	Trapping Sites (Villages) selected
1. Ukusijoni	1. Maaji-Sinyanya-Ofu	*Glossina fuscipes fuscipes,* and *G. morsitans spp.*	1.19	1. Maaji-Sinyanya-Ofu
	2. Kiraba	*Glossina fuscipes fuscipes*	3.80	
	3. Panyawe	*Glossina fuscipes fuscipes*	4.90	2. Panyawe-Kobo
	4. Okangali	*Glossina fuscipes fuscipes*	3.00	
	5. Paeiyaro	*Glossina fuscipes fuscipes*	0.13	
2. Arinyapi	6. Madulu/Itoasi	*Glossina fuscipes fuscipes*	0.03	3. Madulu/Itoasi
	7. Ogolo	Nil	0.00	
	8. Oriangwa/Melehwe	Nil	0.00	
	9. Ovuvu/Pamajua	Nil	0.00	
	10. Nzolohwe/Oniazo	*Glossina fuscipes fuscipes*	0.10	4. Nzolohwe/Oniazo
3. Odu	11. Pakwinya	*Glossina fuscipes fuscipes*	6.80	5. Pakwinya
	12. Odu	*Glossina fuscipes fuscipes*	0.50	6. Odu
	13. Ofua Central	Nil	0.00	
4. Ataboo	14. Ataboo Central	*Glossina fuscipes fuscipes*	0.10	
	15. Palanyua	*Glossina fuscipes fuscipes*	0.30	7. Palanyua
	16. Olia	*Glossina fuscipes fuscipes*	0.10	
	17. Amelo	*Glossina fuscipes fuscipes*	0.20	
	18. Pereci	*Glossina fuscipes fuscipes*	0.10	
	19. Paluga	*Glossina fuscipes fuscipes*	0.50	8. Paluga
5. Palaro	20. Amuru	*Glossina fuscipes fuscipes*	0.15	
	21. Paoja	*Glossina fuscipes fuscipes*	0.20	
	22. Melijo	*Glossina fuscipes fuscipes*	0.50	9. Melijo
	23. Fuda	*Glossina fuscipes fuscipes*	0.11	
	24. Lewa	*Glossina fuscipes fuscipes*	0.33	
	25. Okawa	*Glossina fuscipes fuscipes*	0.44	10. Okawa
	26. Boroli	*Glossina fuscipes fuscipes*	0.06	
6. Paridi	27. Esia	*Glossina fuscipes fuscipes*	15.00	11. Esia (along river Esia)
	28. Openzinzi	Nil	0.00	
	29. Endrebamvuku	Nil	0.00	
	30. Moinya	*Glossina fuscipes fuscipes*	31.00	12. Moinya (along river Itirikwa)
	31. Pakondo	Nil	0.00	
7. Lajopi	32. Unna	Nil	0.00	
	33. Mokolo/Murenica	Nil	0.00	
	34. Rende	Nil	0.00	
Total			69.54	
Average			2.045	

Results of the systematic survey (Tables 3 and IV) indicate that 3 different tsetse fly species exist in Adjumani District, namely *G. f. fuscipes*, *G. m. submorsitans*, and *G. pallidipes*. Overall, out of the total of 1,570 tsetse flies caught during the survey period, *G. f. fuscipes* was the most abundant tsetse species distributed in all the 6 parishes and 12 trapping sites with a total of 1,401 individuals caught, giving an average fly trapping density (FTD) of 1.765; followed by *G. m. submorsitans* found in Maaji-Sinyanya-Ofu Village in Ukusijoni Parish, Okawa Village in Palaro Parish, and Pakwinya Village in Odu Parish with a total of 143 individuals caught, giving an average FTD of 0.174; and the least abundant species being *G. pallidipes* confined to Maaji-Sinyanya-Ofu Village in Ukusijoni Parish, with a total of only 26 individuals caught, giving an average FTD of 0.0308. Comparing between locations and trapping sites, the highest relative percentage composition of *G. f. fuscipes* was registered in Palaro Parish (approximately 32%), followed by Paridi Parish (approximately 22%), with the lowest (about 4%) being registered in Ataboo Parish (Figure 1). Although *G. m. submorsitans* was caught in Okawa Village in Palaro Parish and Pakwinya Village in Odu Parish, the relative percentage composition figures were very negligible in these villages and parishes, compared to that in Maaji-Sinyanya-Ofu Village in Ukusijoni Parish. It appeared to have confined itself again mainly to Maaji-Sinyanya-Ofu Village in Ukusijoni Parish. Ukusijoni Parish therefore had the highest tsetse species diversity. Possibly this distribution pattern of *G. f. fuscipes*, *G. m. submorsitans*, and *G. pallidipes* could have been influenced by the availability of local preferred food sources, as suggested earlier by FAO (1982b) and Minter (1996). Minter (1996) also pointed out that where there is no close contact with man and domestic animals, flies of the *Palpalis group* show a preference of feeding on large reptiles, such as monitor lizards and crocodiles. Probably this explains why *G. f. fuscipes* was caught along river courses where these reptiles are found. Species of the *Morsitans* group obtain most of their blood meals from the wild animals, especially Bovidae and Suidae, that roam the savanna (FAO, 1982b; and Minter, 1996). This could have been the reason for *G. m. submorsitans* and *G. pallidipes* all of *Morsitans* species group to be distributed far away from human settlements in Maaji-Sinyanya-Ofu, Odu, and Okawa villages where the abundance of these wild animals coming from the nearby Zoka Forest is higher. Nevertheless, *G. m. submorsitans* and *G. pallidipes* were still caught along the available river courses in those areas. All the three species of *G. f. fuscipes*, *G. m. submorsitans*, and *G. pallidipes* overlapped in Maaji-Sinyanya-Ofu Village in Ukusijoni Parish with no clear boundary while the 2 species of *G. f. fuscipes* and *G. m. submorsitans* overlapped in Odu Village in Odu Parish and in Okawa Village in Palaro Parish, also without clear boundary.

Table 3: The Number of Tsetse Flies Caught per Site per Location, April – September 2002

Species	Study Locations, Trapping Sites, Total of Individuals Caught												
	Ukusijoni		Arinyapi		Odu		Ataboo		Palaro		Paridi		Total
	M-S-O	P-K	M/I	N/O	Pakwinya	Odu	Palanyua	Paluga	Melijo	Okawa	Esia	Moinya	
G. m. subm.	140	00	00	00	00	01	00	00	00	02	00	00	143
G. f. f.	23	175	57	41	52	162	31	30	314	171	196	149	1,401
G. p.	26	00	00	00	00	00	00	00	00	00	00	00	26

Key: G. m. m. (*Glossina morsitans submorsitans*); G. f. f. (*Glossina fuscipes fuscipes*); G. p. (*Glossina pallidipes*); M-S-O (Maaji-Sinyanya-Ofu Village); P-K (Panyawe-Kobo Village); M/I (Madulu/Itoasi Village); and N/O (Nzolohwe/Oniazo Village)

Table 4: FTD per Site per Location, April – September 2002

Species	Study Locations, Trapping Sites, and Average FTD												
	Ukusijoni		Arinyapi		Odu		Ataboo		Palaro		Paridi		Av.
	M-S-O	P-K	M/I	N/O	Pakwinya	Odu	Palanyua	Paluga	Melijo	Okawa	Esia	Moinya	FTD
G. m. subm.	2.06	00	00	00	00	0.01	00	00	00	0.02	00	00	0.174
G. f. f.	0.37	2.51	1.26	0.65	0.75	2.48	0.46	0.45	4.70	2.39	2.99	2.17	1.765
G. p.	0.37	00	00	00	00	00	00	00	00	00	00	00	0.0308

Key: G. m. m. (*Glossina morsitans submorsitans*); G. f. f. (*Glossina fuscipes fuscipes*); G. p. (*Glossina pallidipes*); M-S-O (Maaji-Sinyanya-Ofu Village); P-K (Panyawe-Kobo Village); M/I (Madulu/Itoasi Village); N/O (Nzolohwe/Oniazo Village); Av. FTD (Average Fly Trapping Density).

As shown in Table 5, the total of 1,570 tsetse flies caught during the survey disaggregated into 416 non-teneral male tsetse flies (26%), 219 teneral male tsetse flies (14%), 637 non-teneral female tsetse flies (41%), and 298 teneral female tsetse flies (19%). Overall, there were 635 males (40%), and 935 females (60%). The higher number of non-teneral female flies compared their counterpart non-teneral males is a recipe for population increase (FAO, 1982b). The monthly tsetse fly catches also indicate that the number of individuals caught for the 2 species of G. f. fuscipes and G. m. submorsitans both increased and decreased simultaneously following more or less the same patterns during the 6 months study period. The numbers simultaneously rose from April and reached their peaks in May, then dropped smoothly to their lowest levels in July, rose sharply and reached their second peaks in August (Figure II), dropping sharply again in September, although G. m. submorsitans tended to maintain a slight rise from July, through August to September.

Table 5: Monthly Tsetse Fly Age and Sex Distribution in Adjumani District, April – September 2002

Age and Sex Category	Months						Total	% Composition
	April	May	June	July	August	September		
NTM	119	122	45	23	75	32	416	26
TM	22	65	24	12	59	37	219	14
NTF	134	200	94	33	117	59	637	41
TF	50	44	33	31	108	32	298	19
TOTAL	325	431	196	99	358	160	1,570	100

Key: NTM (Non-Teneral Males); TM (Teneral Males); NTF (Non-Teneral Females); and TF (Teneral Females).

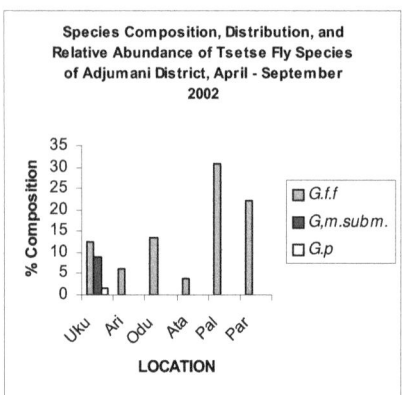

Species Composition, Distribution, and
Relative Abundance of Tsetse Fly Species
of Adjumani District, April - September
2002

% Composition

LOCATION

Key: G.f.f (Glossina fuscipes fuscipes), G,m.subm. (Glossina morsitans submorsitans), G.p (Glossina pallidipes)

Figure 1
Key: G.f.f. (*Glossina fuscipes fuscipes*), *G, m. subm.* (*Glossina morsitans submorsitans*), *G.p* (*Glossina pallidipes*); Uku (Ukusijoni Parish), Ari (Arinyapi Parish), Odu (Odu Parish), Ata (Ataboo Parish), Pal (Palaro Parish), and Par (Paridi Parish).

The catches of *Glossina pallidipes* remained minimal and more or less constant throughout the study period. Probably this simultaneous rise and fall pattern of *G. f. fuscipes* and *G. m. submorsitans* catches was dictated upon by salient environmental factors. For example, as mentioned earlier, the area can be hot during dry season. Worse still, people in the area have developed a habit of burning bush during dry season (November-March), probably for hunting the wild animals mentioned earlier. The bush fires leave the place devoid of vegetation, further increasing the environmental temperature of the area. To escape the high temperatures, many of the wild animals in the area access remote and cooler locations, including hiding in burrows and holes, and would therefore be inaccessible to be fed on by tsetse flies. Many seasonal streams and rivers in the area also dry up during the dry season. A variety of wild host food animals for tsetse flies will collect at the few remaining dry season water points. A lot of human activities also take place at these water points, including fetching water, bathing, fishing, watering domestic animals, and hunting; exposing additional human and domestic animal hosts. All these would have provided food sources plenty enough for tsetse flies to increase in numbers especially during dry season, but this appears not to be the case here. The rising nature in tsetse numbers caught in the month of April reflects that there was probably a decline in their numbers during the previous dry season. This can be attributed to the scorching sun heat and lack of vegetation which also force tsetse flies to resort to hidden and cooler habitats such as the gallery forests, river beds, rot holes, and caves, and become less abundant. This is in agreement with suggestions made by Nash (1969) and FAO (1982b). The bush fires must have killed many individuals, further reducing their numbers.

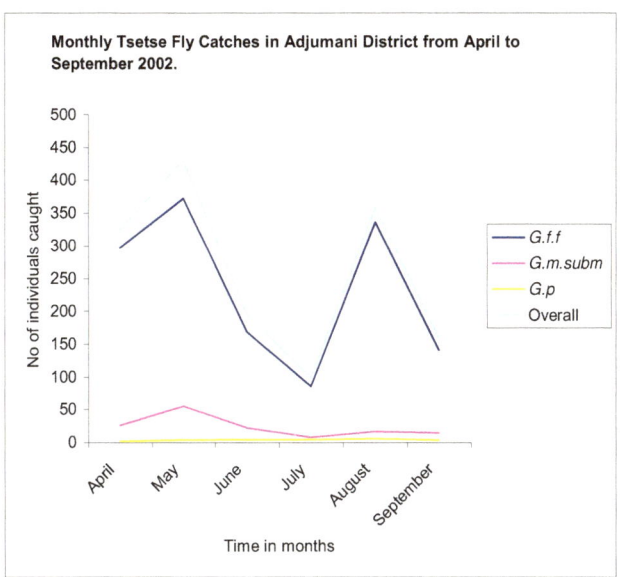

Monthly Tsetse Fly Catches in Adjumani District from April to September 2002.

Time in months

Figure II
Key: *G.f.f.* (*Glossina fuscipes fuscipes*), *G. m. subm.* (*Glossina morsitans submorsitans*), *G.p* (*Glossina pallidipes*)

Environmental temperature, among other factors, appears to have a marked effect on the distribution and abundance of tsetse flies in an area, more or less equal in strength to availability of local preferred food sources, and that probably explains also why low numbers were caught in July following a short dry spell in the month of June. Relatively high numbers were caught in the months of April and May because these were the months when rains had just started in the area and the tsetse flies were emerging from their hideouts. The start of the rains could have also provided suitable conditions for the emergence of adults from pupae, which could have probably been in a dormant state due to the too high temperatures of the previous dry season. The overall picture of the species composition and relative abundance of the different tsetse fly species of Adjumani District is provided in Figure 3, with *G. f. fuscipes* constituting the highest percentage composition (89%), followed by *G. m. submorsitans* (9%), and lastly *G. pallidipes* at 2%.

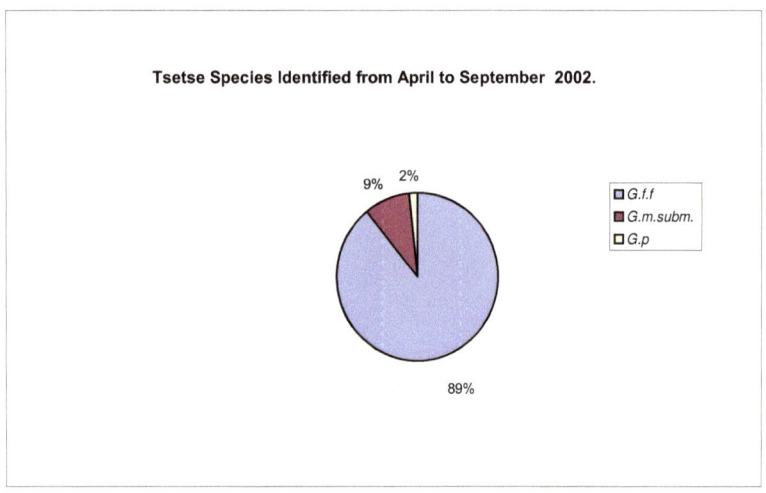

Tsetse Species Identified from April to September 2002.

Key:
- G.f.f
- G.m.subm.
- G.p

9%   2%

89%

Figure 3

Key: G.f.f. (*Glossina fuscipes fuscipes*), G. m. subm. (*Glossina morsitans submorsitans*), G.p (*Glossina pallidipes*)

Tsetse-borne trypanosomiasis problem would be expected to match the number or the species diversity of tsetse flies caught in a location but the results here do not agree. For example, Arinyapi Area had a relative tsetse percentage composition (of G. f. fuscipes only) at approximately 7% (Figure 1), more than 4 times less than that of Palaro Parish (32%), but registered the highest number of sleeping sickness patients admitted in the hospital during the study period (Figure IV). These included Sleeping Sickness Stage II cases. Another area that registered relatively high numbers of Sleeping Sickness cases, including also Stage II cases, was Odu, yet it had tsetse fly percentage composition of less than 15%. Although the percentage composition of G. f. fuscipes tsetse flies caught in Palaro Parish was the highest, only 4 sleeping sickness cases were admitted from that area. Unfortunately, they were all stage II cases (100%). One person was admitted from Ataboo Parish and was also found to be Stage II case of sleeping sickness. 1 person admitted from Ukusijoni Parish, which was the richest in terms of tsetse species diversity, during the study period, was found still at Stage I of the sleeping sickness disease. It is apparent that there is no positive correlation between the number of Sleeping Sickness patients admitted and number and species diversity of tsetse flies caught in a particular area. This could be attributed to the fact that trypanosome infection rate of tsetse flies varies from place to place, species to species, and from time to time (Jordan, 1961; and Jordan, 1965). Perhaps many of the tsetse flies in the high tsetse infested areas like Melijo Village in Palaro Parish, and Paridi Parish are lowly infected, while those in

Arinyapi-Mgbere-Southern-Sudan and Odu-Kureku areas are highly infected. Out of the total of 41 sleeping sickness patients admitted in Adjumani Hospital during the survey period, majority (17) of them came from Arinyapi Area, including Mgbere Parish, and Southern Sudan (Anonymous, 2002c-unpublished). Each month, among the Sleeping Sickness patients admitted in Adjumani Hospital during the survey period, the number of refugees and other people from Southern Sudan was higher than that of Ugandan nationals (Figure 5). The long civil war, lasting at least 20 years, in the Sudan hampered tsetse and trypanosomiasis control operations in Southern Sudan, and as a result there was no control there (Mutumba-Lule, 2001). Trypanosomes could also have been circulating and spreading from Southern Sudan. The Gambian form of sleeping sickness in the area is chronic, slow in its manifestations, and insidious in its onset. In the absence of active screening by government like the case in the area, victims would not normally realize the disease immediately and would take long to go for medical check up in the hospital by themselves (passive screening). By the time the victims decide to go for medical check up, it would be a bit late and the disease would have progressed to that advanced Stage II observed here.

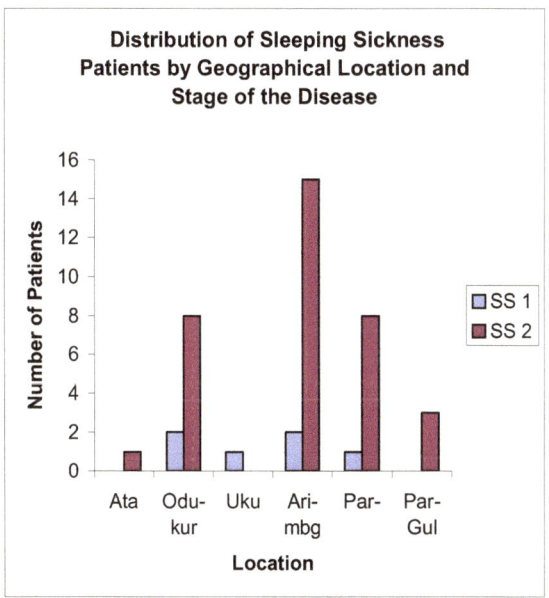

Figure IV
Key: SS 1 (Sleeping Sickness Stage 1); SS 2 (Sleeping Sickness Stage 2); Ata (Ataboo Area); Odu-kur (Odu Area, including Kureku Parish); Uku (Ukusijoni Area); Ari-mbg (Arinyapi Area, including Mgbere Parish and Southern Sudan); Par- (Paridi Area); and Par-Gul (Palaro Area, including Gulu District)

G. *fuscipes fuscipes* of *Palpalis* species group, G. *m. submorsitans* and G. *pallidipes* both of *Morsitans* species group were all found to exist along river courses; hence they all existed as riverine vegetation tsetse, as opposed to the general thought that G. *m. submorsitans* and G. *pallidipes* always exist as open savanna *Acacia-Combretum* vegetation tsetse. However, there are differences in the geographical location of the tsetse flies of Adjumani District. G. *f. fuscipes* was found in all the 6 parishes and 12 trapping sites, while G. *m. submorsitans*, and G. *pallidipes* were found confined mainly to Maaji-Sinyanya-Ofu Village in Ukusijoni Parish, a pattern influenced by salient environmental factors, including availability of preferred local sources of food as explained earlier.

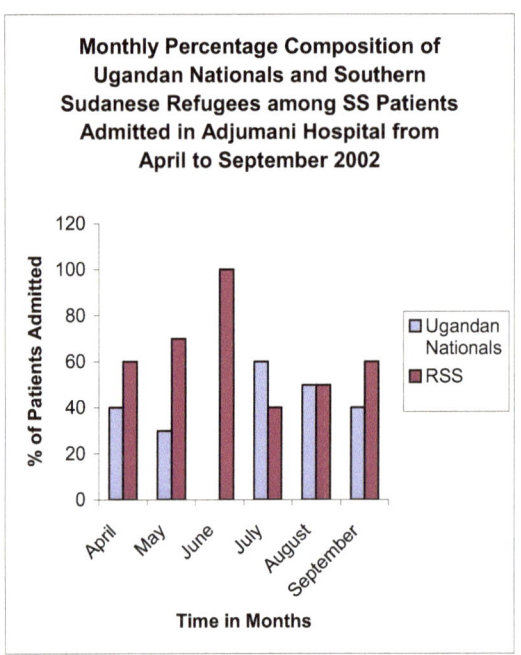

Figure 5
Key: SS (Sleeping Sickness); and RSS (Refugees from Southern Sudan)

18

GENERAL RECOMMENDATIONS: The benefits and the future

Before this research, only one method of tsetse control of setting pyramidal traps only along river banks was used, targeting riverine tsetse, in reaction to sleeping sickness cases reported and complaints received from local communities rather than basing on concrete information on the tsetse species present, their distribution patterns and relative abundance. The research has generated knowledge about the different tsetse species that exist in Adjumani District and their distribution patterns and relative abundance, which should be used to guide future choice and use of the appropriate methods of tsetse control in the district.

The tsetse fly species of Adjumani District have been described and the description of the species has added onto the existing body of scientific knowledge, which should be referred to in future.

The distinguishing features of each of the 3 tsetse fly species found present in Adjumani District have been used to construct identification keys. The identification keys can be used to train new tsetse control personnel in the district in the identification of *Glossina* species or for future research work.

Environmental temperature, among other factors, affects to a great extent the distribution and abundance of tsetse flies in Adjumani District. The corresponding temperature range in the area during dry season should be captured in similar surveys in future for a deeper analysis and understanding.

The availability of local food sources appears to have also partly influenced the distribution patterns of the tsetse fly species studied. Further research is needed to investigate host preference of tsetse flies in the district.

The knowledge generated here is of use to many stakeholders, including governments, universities, students, donors. There is therefore need to upgrade it further and to publish it at Masters or PhD thesis level for a wider publicity; with more data and an in-depth analysis.

CONCLUSION

G. fuscipes fuscipes of *Palpalis* species group, and *G. m. submorsitans* and *G. pallidipes* both of *Morsitans* species group were all found along river courses in riverine vegetation, with *G. m. submorsitans* and *G. pallidipes* confined to Maaji-Sinyanya-Ofu Village in Ukusijoni Parish. Targeted deployment of insecticide treated pyramidal traps along river courses in all the 12 villages and 6 parishes affected by *G. f. fuscipes*, and biconical traps also along river courses mainly in Maaji-Sinyanya-Ofu Village affected by *G. m. submorsitans* and *G. pallidipes* would stop wastage of resources.

Non-teneral female tsetse flies caught were one and a half times more in number than their counterpart non-teneral males. This ratio is too high. Since a male tsetse fly can mate with more than one female, and since old males are better-able to mate successfully than the very young ones, this ratio signifies a salient potential for population increase.

Tsetse flies appear to be weakened by the high temperatures of the dry season. Launching an area-wide attack such as sterile insect technique-SIT or mass rearing and release of a natural enemy or applying an appropriate contact insecticide in their breeding habitats just before the onset of rains would suppress the populations drastically.

The disparities between the number of tsetse flies caught in a particular area and the corresponding number of Sleeping Sickness cases admitted from that area observed here can best be explained by an independent scientific investigation into the trypanosome infection rates of tsetse flies of Adjumani District, which is still wanting.

The sleeping sickness type in Adjumani District is the insidious one and victims take long to realize it and usually they report for medical check late when the disease has already progressed to the advanced stage (Stage II) which is difficult to cure. Resumption of regular mass sensitization and screening programmes would reduce the burden.

The persistent wars in the region have destroyed the systems and structures put in place to contain the tsetse and trypanosomiasis problem in the area, including Southern Sudan. This has in turn led to the rampant Sleeping Sickness epidemic outbreaks reported, and these outbreaks are likely to continue in future in both countries if a bilateral co-operation is not forged towards a long term solution to the problem.

BIBLIOGRAPHY

- ANONYMOUS (2000a). Project of Global 2000 River Blindness Program and Ministry of Health. Vol. 8 No. 12. Kampala.
- ANONYMOUS (2000b-unpublished). Adjumani Hospital Records from October 1999 to March 2000.
- ANONYMOUS (2000c-unpublished). Monthly Tsetse Control Records for the months of March and April, 2000. Department of Entomology, Adjumani District.
- ANONYMOUS (2002a-unpublished). Records from District Population Office Adjumani 2002.
- ANONYMOUS (2002b-unpublished). Records from District Veterinary Office Adjumani 2002.
- ANONYMOUS (2002c-unpublished). Adjumani Hospital Records from April to September 2002.
- BARETT, M. (2001). "Drug Resistance in Sleeping Sickness". Africa Health. Incorporating Medicine Digest. Vol. 23, Number 3.
- BIRYOMUMAISHO, SAVINO. "Trypanosomiasis: A disease of Animals and People". A short Certificate Course in New Techniques in Tsetse and Trypanosomiasis Control. Makerere University Faculty of Veterinary Medicine. Kampala. Uganda. 2007a: p43-49.
- COCTU (1995). Annual Report on Tsetse and Trypanosomiasis Research and Control in Uganda.
- COCTU (1996). Quarterly Report Second Quarter 1996 (April-June 1996).
- COOK, G. (1996). Manson's Tropical Diseases. 20th Edition. W.B Saunders. London.
- DRATELE, C. (1999). The Prevalence of Bovine Trypanosomiasis and the level of Community Participation in Tsetse and Trypanosomiasis Control in Adjumani District. BVM Dissertation, Makerere University, Kampala, Uganda.
- EGADU, S.P. (2000). A Visit to ACCORD Adjumani Program 26th to 28th April 2000. The Trip Report. Head of KPIU Environment and Agriculture Desk.
- FAO (1982a). Training Manual for Tsetse Control Personnel. Vol. 3: Control Methods and Side Effects. FAO. Rome. 128pp.
- FAO (1982b). Training Manual for Tsetse Control Personnel. Vol. 1: Tsetse Biology, Systematics and Distribution Techniques. FAO. Rome. 279pp.
- HURSEY, B.S. (2001). "The Programme Against African Trypanosomiasis (PAAT)". Trends in Parasitology. Elsevier Scie. Ltd.
- JORDAN, A.M. (1961). An Assessment of the economic importance of tsetse species of Southern Nigeria and Southern Cameroon based on their trypanosome infection rates and ecology. Commonwealth Institute of Entomology, London.
- JORDAN, A.M. (1965). "The Hosts of *Glossina* as the Main Factor affecting Trypanosome Infection Rates of Tsetse Flies in Nigeria". Transactions of the Royal Society of Tropical Medicine and Hygiene. Vol. 59. No. 4 pp 423-431.
- LANGDALE-BROWN, OSMASTON, H.A and WILSON, J.G. (1964). The Vegetation of Uganda. Uganda Government Department of Lands and Surveying. Uganda.

- MAAIF (2012). A Technical and Financial Proposal for the Uganda Tsetse & Trypanosomiasis Eradication Programme-UTTEP. September 2012. The Republic of Uganda.
- MINTER, D.M. (1996). "Tsetse Flies (*Glossina*)". Manson's Tropical Diseases. 20th Edition. COOK, G. (editor). W.B Saunders. London.
- MOH (2001). "Press Release". Sunday Vision, 6th May 2001. The New Vision Newspaper. The New Vision Printing and Publishing Corporation. Kampala. Uganda.
- MSF (FRANCE). (1992). Annual Report 1992.
- MUTUMBA-LULE, A. (2001). "Sudan Refugees Blamed for Spread of Sleeping Sickness". The East African Magazine April 16-22, 2001. The Nation Group. Nairobi.
- NASH, T.A.M. (1969). Africa's Bane: The Tsetse fly. Collins. London.
- RWABWOOGO, M.O. (1998). Uganda Districts Information Handbook. Fountain Publishers Ltd. Kampala.
- *SCIENCE* DAILY. Lactating Tsetse Flies Models for Lactating Mammals? (Online). Available at http://www.sciencedaily.com/releases/2012/04/120418162302.htm (Retrieved 23 April 2012).
- SERVICE, M.W. (1980). A guide to Medical Entomology. Macmillan Press Ltd., London.
- SMART, J.; JORDAN, K. and WHITTICK, R. J. (1943). A handbook for the identification of insects of medical importance. British Museum. London.

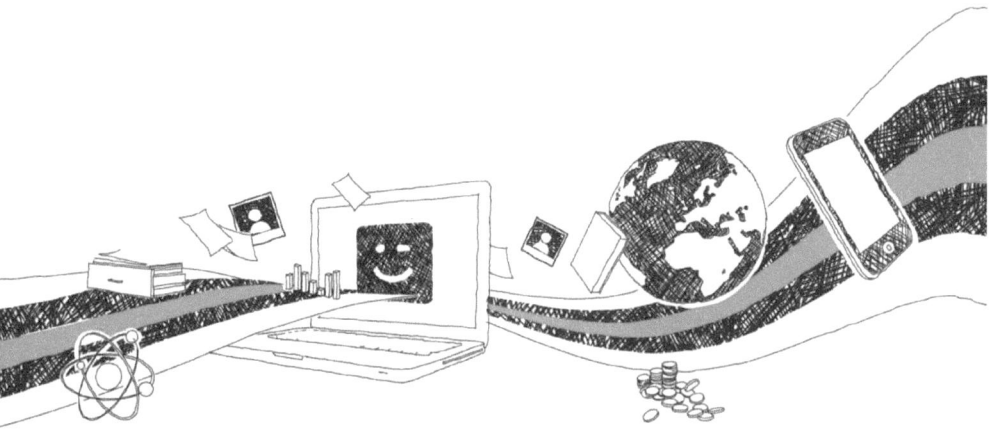
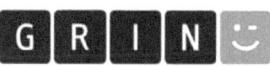